Men's Health Nice Beginners Guide

Understanding Men's Health and Building Healthy Habits

By

Alastair Felix

Table of Contents

CHAPTER 1

Introduction

1.1 The Importance of a Healthy Lifestyle

Maintaining a healthy lifestyle is crucial for men of all ages to enjoy a high quality of life and reduce the risk of developing chronic diseases. A healthy lifestyle encompasses various factors, including regular physical activity, balanced nutrition, stress management, adequate sleep, and avoiding harmful habits. Let's delve deeper into why a healthy lifestyle is essential for men:

1. Promotes Physical Health: Engaging in regular physical activity, such as cardiovascular

exercises, strength training, and flexibility exercises, improves cardiovascular health, boosts the immune system, and helps maintain a healthy weight. Regular exercise also strengthens muscles and bones, reducing the risk of injury and promoting better overall physical function.

2. Reduces the Risk of Chronic Diseases: A healthy lifestyle significantly lowers the risk of developing chronic diseases, such as heart disease, type 2 diabetes, hypertension, and certain types of cancer. By making conscious choices to eat nutritious foods, exercise regularly, and maintain a healthy weight, men can significantly improve their

long-term health outcomes and life expectancy.

3. Supports Mental Well-Being: Physical health and mental well-being are closely interconnected. Engaging in regular exercise releases endorphins, which are natural mood lifters, helping to reduce stress, anxiety, and depression. A balanced diet rich in essential nutrients also supports brain health and cognitive function, enhancing focus and mental clarity.

4. Enhances Sexual Health: Maintaining a healthy lifestyle positively impacts men's sexual health. Regular exercise improves blood circulation, which can contribute to better erectile function. A balanced

diet that includes essential nutrients can also support reproductive health and hormone balance.

5. Boosts Energy Levels: A healthy lifestyle provides the necessary fuel for the body, ensuring sustained energy levels throughout the day. Proper nutrition and regular physical activity improve stamina and productivity, enabling men to perform daily tasks efficiently and stay mentally alert.

6. Improves Sleep Quality: Establishing healthy lifestyle habits, such as adhering to a consistent sleep schedule and reducing stimulants like caffeine and electronic device usage before bedtime, promotes

better sleep quality. Quality sleep is essential for overall health and well-being, as it allows the body to recover and rejuvenate.

7. Enhances Longevity: Studies consistently show that individuals who adopt a healthy lifestyle tend to live longer and enjoy a higher quality of life in their later years. By prioritizing health and wellness, men can increase their chances of living an active and fulfilling life well into their golden years.

8. Serves as a Role Model: Adopting a healthy lifestyle not only benefits the individual but also sets a positive example for friends, family, and the community. As men prioritize their health, they inspire those

around them to do the same, creating a ripple effect of healthier behaviors and improved well-being.

Embracing a healthy lifestyle is a vital step for men to maintain their physical, mental, and emotional well-being. Through regular physical activity, balanced nutrition, and mindful self-care, men can reduce the risk of chronic diseases, boost their energy levels, enhance their sexual health, and improve their overall quality of life. Remember, small, consistent changes can lead to significant improvements in health over time, so start taking steps towards a healthier lifestyle today.

1.2 Setting Realistic Goals

Setting realistic goals is a fundamental aspect of any journey towards better health and well-being. Without clear and achievable objectives, it becomes challenging to stay motivated and track progress effectively. When it comes to men's health, setting realistic goals is crucial for maintaining long-term commitment and avoiding feelings of frustration or disappointment. Here's a guide on how to set realistic goals for your health:

1. Assess Your Current Situation: Before setting goals, take an honest and objective assessment of your current health status. Identify areas that need improvement and areas where you're already doing

well. Consider factors such as physical fitness, nutrition, stress levels, sleep quality, and any existing health conditions. Understanding your starting point will help you set appropriate and achievable objectives.

2. Make Specific Goals: Vague goals are challenging to measure and achieve. Instead, make your objectives specific and well-defined. For example, rather than saying, "I want to get healthier," set a specific goal like, "I will exercise for 30 minutes, five days a week," or "I will eat five servings of fruits and vegetables every day."

3. Set Measurable Targets: Having measurable goals allows you to track your

progress and stay motivated. Use quantifiable metrics to gauge your achievements. For instance, if your goal is to lose weight, set a target of losing a certain number of pounds over a specific period. Measuring your progress helps you stay on course and make adjustments when necessary.

4. Set Realistic and Attainable Goals: While it's essential to challenge yourself, setting unrealistic goals can lead to discouragement and a sense of failure. Be honest about your abilities and limitations. Consider your daily commitments, lifestyle, and any health conditions when determining what you can realistically achieve. Setting

small, incremental goals that you can achieve over time can be more effective than aiming for drastic changes.

5. Create Time-Bound Objectives: Give yourself a timeframe to achieve your goals. Having a deadline creates a sense of urgency and helps you stay focused on your objectives. Setting short-term and long-term goals can provide a clear roadmap for your health journey, allowing you to celebrate small wins along the way.

6. Be Flexible and Adaptable: Life is full of unexpected challenges, and it's essential to be adaptable when it comes to goal-setting. If you encounter obstacles or setbacks, don't be

discouraged. Instead, reassess your goals, make necessary adjustments, and continue moving forward. Being flexible allows you to maintain momentum even in the face of challenges.

7. Celebrate Your Achievements: Recognize and celebrate your progress, no matter how small. Acknowledging your successes boosts your motivation and reinforces positive behavior. Reward yourself for reaching milestones, whether it's treating yourself to something you enjoy or simply taking a moment to reflect on your accomplishments.

8. Seek Support and Accountability: Share your health goals with friends,

family, or a support group.
Having a support system can
provide encouragement,
guidance, and accountability.
Consider working with a health
professional, such as a personal
trainer or a nutritionist, to
create a tailored plan and
receive expert guidance.

Setting realistic goals is not about
perfection; it's about progress and
continuous improvement. Embrace
the journey, be patient with yourself,
and celebrate every step towards
better men's health. By setting
achievable goals, you pave the way
for positive and sustainable changes
that will benefit your overall well-
being in the long run.

CHAPTER 2

Understanding Men's Health

2.1 Key Health Concerns for Men

Men face specific health concerns that are unique to their gender. Understanding and addressing these key health concerns are essential for maintaining optimal well-being. Here are some of the primary health concerns for men:

1. Cardiovascular Disease: Heart disease, including conditions like coronary artery disease, heart attacks, and stroke, is a leading cause of death among

men. Risk factors include high blood pressure, high cholesterol levels, smoking, obesity, and a sedentary lifestyle.

2. Prostate Health: Prostate issues, such as benign prostatic hyperplasia (BPH) and prostate cancer, become more common as men age. Regular prostate screenings and early detection are crucial for successful treatment.

3. Testicular Health: Testicular cancer is the most common cancer among young men. Self-examinations and regular check-ups with a healthcare provider can aid in early detection and improved outcomes.

4. Erectile Dysfunction: Erectile dysfunction (ED) is the inability to achieve or maintain an erection sufficient for sexual intercourse. It can be caused by physical or psychological factors and may be an early indicator of cardiovascular issues.

5. Mental Health: Men can face challenges in addressing mental health concerns due to societal expectations surrounding masculinity. Depression, anxiety, and stress-related disorders are prevalent among men and require attention and support.

6. Type 2 Diabetes: Men are at a higher risk of developing type 2 diabetes, especially if they have a family history of the

condition, are overweight, or lead a sedentary lifestyle.

7. Lung Cancer: Smoking remains a significant risk factor for lung cancer, and men have historically had higher smoking rates. Quitting smoking and avoiding exposure to secondhand smoke are essential for reducing this risk.

8. Colorectal Cancer: Colorectal cancer affects both men and women, but men have a slightly higher risk. Regular screenings, such as colonoscopies, are vital for early detection and successful treatment.

9. Osteoporosis: While osteoporosis is often associated with women, men can also develop this condition,

particularly as they age.
Adequate calcium intake,
vitamin D, and weight-bearing
exercises can help maintain
bone health.

10. Accidents and Injuries: Men are
more likely to engage in risky
behaviors and occupations that
may lead to accidents and
injuries. Taking appropriate
safety precautions and wearing
protective gear can help reduce
the risk.

2.2 Common Health Issues and Risks

Aside from the key health concerns
mentioned above, men also face a
range of common health issues and

risks that can impact their well-being. These may include:

1. Obesity and Overweight: Unhealthy eating habits, sedentary lifestyles, and lack of exercise can contribute to obesity and overweight issues, which are associated with an increased risk of various health problems.

2. Hypertension: High blood pressure is a prevalent health issue among men, and if left untreated, it can lead to serious complications such as heart disease, stroke, and kidney problems.

3. Substance Abuse: Men have higher rates of substance abuse, including alcohol and illicit drugs. Substance abuse can lead

to physical and mental health problems and negatively impact relationships and work performance.

4. Sleep Disorders: Sleep apnea and other sleep disorders are more common in men and can affect overall health and daytime functioning.

5. Injuries in Sports and Physical Activities: Active men participating in sports and physical activities may be prone to injuries, ranging from minor sprains to more severe fractures or ligament tears.

6. Work-Related Stress: Men may face additional stress due to demanding work environments, which can lead to burnout and

negative effects on mental and physical health.

7. Sexual Health Issues: In addition to erectile dysfunction, men may encounter other sexual health issues, such as premature ejaculation or reduced libido, which can impact their overall well-being and relationships.

8. Skin Cancer: Men are more likely to spend time outdoors without proper sun protection, putting them at a higher risk of developing skin cancer.

Understanding these common health issues and risks allows men to be proactive in their approach to health and well-being. Regular medical check-ups, adopting healthy lifestyle habits, seeking support for mental health concerns, and staying informed about preventive measures are essential steps to promote a long and healthy life.

2.3 Age-Related Health Considerations

As men age, their bodies go through various physiological changes that can impact their health and well-being. Understanding and addressing age-related health considerations are crucial for promoting healthy aging and maintaining a high quality of life. Here are some key age-related health considerations for men at different stages of life:

1. Young Adulthood (20s to 30s):

- Establishing Healthy Habits: Young adulthood is an ideal

time to establish healthy lifestyle habits, including regular exercise, a balanced diet, and avoiding harmful behaviors like smoking and excessive alcohol consumption.

- Sexual Health: Young men should practice safe sex, undergo regular testing for sexually transmitted infections (STIs), and consider vaccination for conditions like human papillomavirus (HPV).

- Mental Health: The stress of transitioning into adulthood and building careers can impact mental health. Managing stress and seeking support for any mental health concerns are essential.

- Injury Prevention: Young adults are often more physically active and may engage in sports and recreational activities. Taking precautions to prevent injuries is vital to maintain long-term physical health.

2. Middle Adulthood (40s to 50s):

- Cardiovascular Health: Middle age is a critical time to prioritize cardiovascular health, as the risk of heart disease and hypertension increases. Regular health check-ups and screenings for conditions like high blood pressure and cholesterol are essential.

- Prostate Health: Prostate health becomes a more significant concern in middle age. Regular prostate exams and screenings are crucial for early detection of any issues.

- Weight Management: Metabolism tends to slow down with age, making weight management more challenging. Maintaining a healthy weight through diet and exercise can reduce the risk of various health conditions.

- Bone Health: Men should pay attention to their bone health, as the risk of osteoporosis increases with age. Adequate calcium intake and weight-bearing exercises can help maintain bone density.

3. Late Adulthood (60s and beyond):

- Preventive Health Care: Regular health check-ups and

screenings become even more critical in late adulthood to catch potential health issues early and maintain overall well-being.

- Cognitive Health: Aging can be accompanied by cognitive changes, but regular mental stimulation, a healthy diet, and social engagement can support cognitive function.

- Mobility and Balance: Physical activity, including exercises that promote balance and flexibility, can help maintain mobility and reduce the risk of falls.

- Social Support: Staying socially connected and maintaining meaningful relationships can have positive effects on mental and emotional health.

- Chronic Disease Management: For those with chronic health conditions, proper management and adherence to medical treatments become essential for maintaining health and preventing complications.

Throughout all stages of life, men should be attentive to their health and proactive in seeking medical advice when necessary. Engaging in regular physical activity, adopting a balanced and nutritious diet, managing stress, and staying informed about age-specific health concerns can contribute to healthy aging and a higher quality of life. Taking a holistic approach to health will empower men to enjoy their lives fully, regardless of their age.

CHAPTER 3

Exercise for men

3.1 Starting a Workout Routine

Starting a workout routine as a beginner can be both exciting and intimidating. However, with the right approach and mindset, it can become a rewarding and empowering journey towards improved fitness and overall health. Here are some essential tips for beginners looking to start a workout routine:

1. Set Realistic Goals: Begin by setting achievable and realistic fitness goals. Whether it's increasing endurance, losing weight, building muscle, or

simply improving overall fitness, having clear goals will help you stay motivated and focused.

2. Choose Activities You Enjoy: Find physical activities or exercises that you genuinely enjoy. This could be anything from walking, jogging, cycling, dancing, swimming, or participating in sports. Enjoying the activity will make it easier to stick to your routine.

3. Start Slowly: As a beginner, it's crucial to start slowly and gradually increase the intensity and duration of your workouts. Pushing yourself too hard at the beginning may lead to injuries or burnout. Listen to your body and give it time to adapt.

4. Warm-up and Cool Down: Always warm up before exercising to prepare your muscles and joints for the workout. Afterward, cool down with gentle stretches to improve flexibility and reduce the risk of muscle soreness.

5. Incorporate Rest Days: Rest days are just as important as exercise days. They allow your body to recover and repair itself. Aim for at least one or two rest days per week.

6. Stay Hydrated: Drink plenty of water before, during, and after your workouts to stay hydrated and support optimal performance.

7. Use Proper Form: When performing exercises, focus on

using proper form to prevent injuries and maximize the effectiveness of the workout. If you're unsure, consider seeking guidance from a fitness professional.

8. Listen to Your Body: Pay attention to how your body feels during and after workouts. If you experience pain or discomfort, stop and consult a healthcare provider or fitness expert if needed.

3.2 Cardiovascular Exercises for Men

Cardiovascular exercises, also known as aerobic exercises, are essential for improving cardiovascular health, burning calories, and increasing overall endurance. Here are some popular cardiovascular exercises for men:

1. Running or Jogging: Running or jogging is an excellent way to get your heart rate up and burn calories. Start at a comfortable pace and gradually increase your speed and distance over time.

2. Cycling: Whether on a stationary bike or a road bike, cycling is a low-impact exercise that provides a great cardiovascular workout.

3. Swimming: Swimming is a full-body workout that is gentle on the joints, making it ideal for individuals with joint issues.

4. Jumping Rope: Jumping rope is
    a fun and effective way to
    improve cardiovascular fitness
    and coordination.

5. Dancing: Dancing is not only a
    fun and social activity but also
    a fantastic cardio workout. Join
    a dance class or simply dance
    to your favorite music at home.

6. HIIT (High-Intensity Interval
    Training): HIIT involves short
    bursts of intense exercise
    followed by brief rest periods.
    It can be an efficient way to
    improve cardiovascular fitness
    and burn calories in a shorter
    amount of time.

3.3 Strength Training and Muscle Building

Strength training is essential for building muscle, increasing strength, and improving overall body composition. It's not just for bodybuilders; it benefits people of all ages and fitness levels. Here are some tips for incorporating strength training into your fitness routine:

1. Start with Bodyweight Exercises: Begin with bodyweight exercises like push-ups, squats, lunges, and planks to build a foundation of strength.

2. Use Proper Technique: Focus on using proper form during strength exercises to prevent injuries and target the intended muscle groups effectively.

3. Gradually Increase Resistance: As you become more comfortable with bodyweight exercises, you can progress to using resistance bands, dumbbells, kettlebells, or weight machines to add more challenge.

4. Target Major Muscle Groups: Include exercises that target major muscle groups, such as chest, back, legs, shoulders, and core, in your workout routine.

5. Allow for Rest and Recovery: Muscles need time to recover and grow stronger. Aim for at least 48 hours of rest between strength training sessions for each muscle group.

6. Mix Up Your Routine: Vary your exercises and routines to

keep your workouts interesting
and to challenge different
muscle groups.

7. Consult a Professional: If
    you're new to strength training,
    consider working with a fitness
    trainer or coach who can create
    a personalized program and
    guide you through proper
    techniques.

By incorporating cardiovascular
exercises and strength training into
your fitness routine, you can improve
your overall physical fitness, boost
your energy levels, and enhance your
well-being as a beginner on the path
to a healthier lifestyle. Remember to
listen to your body, stay consistent,
and have fun while challenging
yourself to reach new fitness goals.

3.4 Flexibility and Mobility Exercises

Flexibility and mobility exercises are essential components of a well-rounded fitness routine. They can help improve joint range of motion, reduce the risk of injury, enhance posture, and promote better overall movement. Whether you are an athlete, fitness enthusiast, or someone looking to maintain flexibility as you age, incorporating these exercises into your routine can bring numerous benefits. Here are some effective flexibility and mobility exercises:

1. Dynamic Stretching: Dynamic stretching involves moving the muscles and joints through their full range of motion in a controlled manner. It helps

increase blood flow and prepares the body for physical activity. Examples of dynamic stretches include leg swings, arm circles, walking lunges, and hip circles.

2. Static Stretching: Static stretching involves holding a stretch for a prolonged period to lengthen the muscles and improve flexibility. Focus on major muscle groups such as hamstrings, quadriceps, calves, chest, shoulders, and back. Hold each stretch for 15-30 seconds and repeat for 2-3 sets.

3. Yoga: Yoga is an excellent practice for improving flexibility, balance, and overall body awareness. Various yoga poses target different muscle groups and can help release

tension and increase range of motion. Incorporate poses like downward dog, warrior, pigeon, and cobra into your routine.

4. Foam Rolling: Foam rolling, also known as self-myofascial release, uses a foam roller to release muscle knots and improve tissue flexibility. Roll slowly over tight areas, applying gentle pressure, and pause on tender spots for 20-30 seconds.

5. Pilates: Pilates focuses on core strength, stability, and flexibility. It involves controlled movements that engage multiple muscle groups simultaneously, promoting better alignment and mobility.

6. Tai Chi: Tai Chi is a Chinese martial art that emphasizes slow, gentle movements and deep breathing. It can improve balance, coordination, and flexibility while reducing stress.

7. Mobility Drills: Mobility drills are exercises that specifically target joint mobility and can help maintain or improve joint function. Examples include shoulder circles, hip rotations, and ankle circles.

8. Resistance Band Exercises: Using resistance bands can enhance stretching and provide additional resistance to improve flexibility. Incorporate band-assisted stretches for both upper and lower body muscle groups.

9. Neck and Spine Stretches: To maintain good posture and alleviate tension in the neck and back, perform neck rotations, lateral neck stretches, and gentle twists for the spine.

10. Cool-Down Stretches: After a workout, incorporate cool-down stretches to help relax the muscles and prevent stiffness. Focus on the muscles you've targeted during your exercise session.

Flexibility and mobility training should be performed at a comfortable level, and gradual progress is key to preventing injury. Avoid bouncing during stretches, as this can cause muscle strain. Make flexibility and mobility exercises a regular part of your fitness routine, and over time, you'll experience increased joint range of motion, improved muscle flexibility, and enhanced overall movement capabilities.

CHAPTER 4
Mental Well-Being

4.1 Understanding Mental Health

Understanding mental health is crucial for promoting overall well-being and addressing any mental health challenges that may arise. Mental health refers to our emotional, psychological, and social well-being, and it affects how we think, feel, and act. Here are some key points to consider when understanding mental health:

1. Mental Health is a Continuum: Mental health exists on a spectrum, ranging from optimal well-being to mental health

challenges or disorders. Just like physical health, everyone experiences fluctuations in their mental health at different times in life.

2. Mental Health Stigma: Unfortunately, there is still stigma surrounding mental health, which can prevent people from seeking help or discussing their struggles openly. It's essential to break down these barriers and create a supportive environment for mental health discussions.

3. Common Mental Health Disorders: Mental health disorders, such as depression, anxiety, bipolar disorder, and schizophrenia, are common and can affect anyone regardless of age, gender, or background.

4. Risk Factors and Protective Factors: Various factors can influence mental health, including genetics, life experiences, trauma, social support, and coping skills. Identifying protective factors and building resilience can help mitigate the impact of risk factors.

5. Seeking Help: Just like physical health conditions, mental health challenges are treatable. It's essential to seek professional help if you or someone you know is experiencing persistent emotional difficulties or behavioral changes.

6. Holistic Approach: Taking care of mental health involves a holistic approach, including self-care, positive relationships,

stress management, and seeking professional support when needed.

4.2 Managing Stress and Anxiety

Stress and anxiety are common experiences in modern life, but excessive or prolonged stress can negatively impact mental and physical health. Learning to manage stress and anxiety effectively is essential for promoting mental well-being. Here are some strategies to cope with stress and anxiety:

1. Identify Triggers: Recognize the specific situations or factors that trigger stress or anxiety. Awareness helps you develop

coping mechanisms tailored to those triggers.

2. Practice Mindfulness: Mindfulness involves being fully present in the moment without judgment. Techniques like meditation, deep breathing, and yoga can help reduce stress and promote relaxation.

3. Physical Activity: Regular exercise is a powerful stress reliever. Engage in activities you enjoy, such as walking, jogging, dancing, or cycling, to release tension and boost mood-enhancing endorphins.

4. Time Management: Organize your daily tasks and prioritize what needs to be done. Effective time management can

reduce feelings of overwhelm and create a sense of control.

5. Reach Out for Support: Share your feelings with friends, family, or a mental health professional. Talking about your stressors can provide perspective and emotional support.

6. Limit News and Media Consumption: Constant exposure to distressing news can increase anxiety. Set boundaries for media consumption and focus on positive and uplifting content.

7. Establish Boundaries: Learn to say no to additional commitments when you feel overwhelmed. Setting healthy

boundaries protects your time and energy.

8. Consider Relaxation Techniques: Explore relaxation techniques like progressive muscle relaxation, aromatherapy, or taking soothing baths to unwind and reduce stress.

4.3 Tips for Improving Sleep Quality

Sleep plays a vital role in mental well-being, physical health, and overall functioning. Poor sleep quality can negatively impact mood, cognitive function, and overall health. Here are some tips for improving sleep quality:

1. Maintain a Sleep Schedule: Try to go to bed and wake up at the

same time every day, even on weekends. Consistency helps regulate the body's internal clock.

2. Create a Relaxing Bedtime Routine: Establish a calming pre-sleep routine to signal to your body that it's time to wind down. This may include reading, practicing relaxation techniques, or listening to soothing music.

3. Limit Screen Time Before Bed: Avoid using electronic devices such as smartphones, tablets, or computers at least an hour before bedtime. The blue light emitted by these devices can disrupt sleep.

4. Create a Comfortable Sleep Environment: Ensure your

bedroom is conducive to sleep -
a cool, dark, and quiet
environment can promote better
sleep quality.

5. Avoid Heavy Meals and
    Caffeine Close to Bedtime:
    Refrain from consuming large
    meals, caffeine, or stimulants
    close to bedtime, as they can
    interfere with sleep.

6. Limit Daytime Naps: While
    short naps can be beneficial,
    excessive daytime napping may
    disrupt nighttime sleep. Keep
    naps brief and avoid napping
    late in the day.

7. Get Regular Physical Activity:
    Engaging in regular exercise
    can help improve sleep quality,
    but avoid vigorous exercise
    close to bedtime.

8. Manage Stress and Anxiety:
    Implement stress management
    techniques, such as mindfulness
    and relaxation exercises, to
    reduce racing thoughts and
    promote better sleep.

Improving mental well-being and
sleep quality is an ongoing process.
It's essential to be patient with
yourself and implement these
strategies consistently. If sleep
disturbances or mental health
challenges persist, consider seeking
guidance from a healthcare provider
or mental health professional for
personalized support and solutions.

4.4 Building Resilience and Coping Strategies

Building resilience and coping strategies are essential for navigating life's challenges and maintaining mental well-being. Resilience refers to the ability to bounce back from difficult situations, adapt to changes, and thrive in the face of adversity. Developing coping strategies empowers individuals to effectively manage stress, cope with emotions, and maintain a positive outlook on life. Here are some tips to build resilience and cultivate coping strategies:

1. Develop a Support System: Surround yourself with supportive and understanding individuals who can offer encouragement, empathy, and a listening ear during tough

times. Social support is a significant factor in building resilience.

2. Practice Positive Thinking: Cultivate an optimistic outlook by focusing on the positives and reframing negative thoughts. Engage in positive self-talk and challenge negative assumptions about yourself and the situation.

3. Embrace Change: Accept that change is a natural part of life, and see challenges as opportunities for growth and learning. Being flexible and adaptable can help you navigate uncertainties with greater ease.

4. Set Realistic Goals: Set achievable and realistic goals that align with your values and

aspirations. Celebrate progress,
no matter how small, and use
setbacks as learning
experiences rather than failures.

5. Practice Mindfulness:
   Mindfulness techniques, such
   as meditation and deep
   breathing, can help you stay
   present in the moment, reduce
   stress, and increase self-
   awareness.

6. Engage in Regular Physical
   Activity: Exercise not only
   benefits physical health but also
   has positive effects on mental
   well-being. It releases
   endorphins, which are natural
   mood boosters, and reduces
   stress.

7. Seek Professional Help: If you
   encounter significant

challenges or find it difficult to cope, don't hesitate to seek guidance from a mental health professional. They can offer valuable insights and support tailored to your individual needs.

8. Build Problem-Solving Skills: Enhance your problem-solving skills to tackle challenges more effectively. Break problems down into smaller steps and consider potential solutions.

9. Engage in Relaxation Techniques: Engaging in relaxation activities like yoga, tai chi, or spending time in nature can help you unwind, reduce stress, and promote emotional well-being.

10. Cultivate Self-Compassion: Treat yourself with kindness and compassion, especially during difficult times. Be gentle with yourself and avoid self-criticism.

11. Learn from Past Experiences: Reflect on past experiences and the coping strategies that worked well for you. Drawing from past successes can build confidence and resilience in current challenges.

12. Practice Gratitude: Regularly express gratitude for the positive aspects of your life. Gratitude exercises can shift focus from difficulties to the blessings in your life.

Building resilience and coping strategies takes time and practice.

Embrace a growth mindset, be patient with yourself, and remember that resilience is a skill that can be developed and strengthened over time. By incorporating these strategies into your life, you can better navigate stress, adversity, and uncertainty, fostering greater mental well-being and a more positive outlook on life.

CHAPTER 5

Preventive Health Measures

5.1 Regular Health Check-ups and Screenings

Regular health check-ups and screenings are vital components of preventive healthcare. They involve routine visits to healthcare professionals, such as primary care doctors, to assess overall health and detect potential health issues early. Here are some key aspects of regular health check-ups and screenings:

1. Frequency: Depending on your age, health status, and risk

factors, you should schedule regular check-ups with your healthcare provider. Typically, adults should have a comprehensive check-up at least once a year.

2. Comprehensive Physical Examination: During a check-up, your healthcare provider will conduct a thorough physical examination, checking vital signs, evaluating organ systems, and assessing overall health.

3. Health Risk Assessment: Your healthcare provider will discuss your lifestyle, medical history, family history, and any potential risk factors to determine appropriate preventive measures.

4. Blood Pressure Measurement: Regular blood pressure monitoring is essential for detecting hypertension, which is a significant risk factor for cardiovascular disease.

5. Cholesterol Testing: Screening for cholesterol levels helps assess cardiovascular risk and informs lifestyle and treatment recommendations.

6. Blood Glucose Testing: Blood glucose screening is important for detecting diabetes or pre-diabetes, which can be managed effectively with early intervention.

7. Cancer Screenings: Depending on age and risk factors, cancer screenings such as mammograms, colonoscopies,

and prostate-specific antigen (PSA) tests are recommended for early detection of certain cancers.

8. Immunizations: Ensuring that vaccinations are up-to-date is crucial for preventing vaccine-preventable diseases and protecting public health.

5.2 Vaccinations and Immunizations

Vaccinations and immunizations are among the most effective preventive health measures available. They protect individuals and communities from infectious diseases by stimulating the immune system to produce antibodies against specific pathogens. Here are some essential points regarding vaccinations and immunizations:

1. Childhood Vaccinations: Childhood vaccination schedules are designed to protect children from various diseases, including measles, mumps, rubella, polio, hepatitis, and more. Following the recommended vaccination schedule is critical for maintaining herd immunity and preventing outbreaks.

2. Adult Vaccinations: Immunizations are not just for children. Adults should stay up-to-date on vaccinations, including those for influenza, pneumococcal disease, tetanus, diphtheria, pertussis, and others.

3. Travel Vaccinations: If you're
    traveling to areas with specific
    health risks, consult with a
    travel health specialist to
    receive appropriate
    vaccinations for the destination.

4. Boosters and Catch-Up
    Vaccinations: Some
    vaccinations require booster
    shots to maintain immunity
    over time. Additionally,
    individuals who missed certain
    vaccinations earlier in life may
    need catch-up vaccinations.

5. Herd Immunity: Vaccinations
    not only protect the vaccinated
    individual but also contribute to
    herd immunity. When a
    significant portion of a
    population is vaccinated, it
    helps prevent the spread of
    diseases and protects those who

cannot be vaccinated, such as those with compromised immune systems.

5.3 Understanding Family Medical History

Understanding your family medical history is essential for assessing your risk of developing certain health conditions. Many diseases, such as heart disease, diabetes, certain cancers, and genetic disorders, can have a hereditary component. Here's why understanding family medical history is important:

1. Risk Assessment: Family medical history helps identify patterns of certain health conditions in your family tree,

providing insights into potential health risks you may face.

2. Preventive Measures: Armed with knowledge about your family medical history, you can take proactive steps to prevent or manage conditions that may run in your family.

3. Screening Recommendations: Based on your family medical history, your healthcare provider may recommend specific screenings or tests to detect conditions early, when they are most treatable.

4. Genetic Counseling: If certain genetic disorders are present in your family, genetic counseling can provide information about inheritance patterns and options for family planning.

5. Informing Healthcare
    Providers: Make sure to share
    your family medical history
    with your healthcare providers
    during check-ups and
    screenings to help them tailor
    preventive care and screenings
    to your specific needs.

6. Family Health Discussions:
    Open conversations about
    family medical history can
    encourage relatives to share
    important health information,
    fostering a collective effort to
    prioritize preventive healthcare.

Preventive health measures are
essential for maintaining well-being
and preventing the onset or
progression of many health
conditions. Regular health check-ups,
vaccinations, and understanding
family medical history are powerful

tools for taking control of your health and promoting a healthier and happier life.

5.4 Lifestyle Choices for Long-term Health

Lifestyle choices play a significant role in determining our long-term health and well-being. Making positive lifestyle changes can prevent chronic diseases, improve overall health, and enhance quality of life. Here are some essential lifestyle choices to consider for long-term health:

1. Balanced and Nutritious Diet:

- Consume a variety of fruits, vegetables, whole grains, lean proteins, and healthy fats.

- Limit intake of processed foods, sugary drinks, and excessive salt.

- Stay hydrated by drinking plenty of water throughout the day.

2. Regular Physical Activity:

- Engage in regular exercise, including aerobic activities, strength training, and flexibility exercises.

- Aim for at least 150 minutes of moderate-intensity exercise or 75 minutes of vigorous-intensity exercise per week, as recommended by health guidelines.

3. Adequate Sleep:

- Prioritize sleep and aim for 7-9 hours of quality sleep each night.

- Establish a consistent sleep schedule and create a relaxing bedtime routine.

4. Avoid Smoking and Limit Alcohol:

- Quit smoking or avoid exposure to tobacco smoke to reduce the risk of numerous health conditions.

- Limit alcohol consumption and follow recommended guidelines for moderate drinking, if you choose to drink.

5. Manage Stress:

- Practice stress management techniques such as mindfulness, deep breathing, yoga, or meditation.

- Engage in hobbies and activities that bring joy and relaxation.

6. Maintain a Healthy Weight:

- Strive for a healthy weight based on your body mass index (BMI) and maintain it through a balanced diet and regular exercise.

7. Stay Hydrated:

- Drink sufficient water daily to stay hydrated and support bodily functions.

8. Practice Safe Sun Exposure:

- Protect your skin from harmful UV rays by using sunscreen, wearing protective clothing, and seeking shade when outdoors.

9. Regular Health Check-ups:

- Schedule regular check-ups with healthcare providers to monitor your health and catch potential issues early.

10. Avoid Substance Abuse:

- Avoid the use of illicit drugs and misuse of prescription medications.

- Seek help if you or someone you know is struggling with substance abuse.

11. Social Connections:

- Cultivate strong social connections with friends, family, and community to support mental and emotional well-being.

12. Mental Health Care:

- Prioritize mental health by seeking support from therapists, counselors, or mental health professionals when needed.

- Practice self-care and stress reduction techniques to promote mental well-being.

Remember that small, consistent lifestyle changes can lead to significant long-term health benefits. Choose one or two areas to focus on initially, and gradually incorporate more healthy habits into your daily routine. Making these positive lifestyle choices can contribute to a healthier, happier, and more fulfilling life as you age.

CHAPTER 6
Men's Sexual Health

6.1 Maintaining Sexual Health and Vitality

Maintaining sexual health and vitality is essential for overall well-being and quality of life. Sexual health encompasses physical, emotional, mental, and social aspects of sexuality. Here are some tips to promote men's sexual health and vitality:

1. Communication: Open and honest communication with your partner about sexual desires, concerns, and preferences fosters a healthy sexual relationship.

2. Safe Sex: Practicing safe sex, including using condoms and getting tested regularly for sexually transmitted infections (STIs), is crucial for sexual health.

3. Regular Exercise: Regular physical activity improves blood circulation, stamina, and mood, which can positively impact sexual function.

4. Balanced Diet: A healthy diet rich in nutrients can support sexual health by promoting hormonal balance and overall well-being.

5. Manage Stress: Chronic stress can negatively affect libido and sexual function. Stress management techniques like

relaxation exercises and mindfulness can be beneficial.

6. Limit Alcohol and Substance Use: Excessive alcohol and drug use can impair sexual performance and decrease sexual desire.

7. Get Enough Sleep: Prioritize sufficient sleep to support hormone production and overall vitality.

8. Avoid Smoking: Smoking can impair blood flow and damage blood vessels, potentially affecting erectile function.

9. Stay Hydrated: Drinking enough water helps maintain overall health, including sexual function.

10. Regular Check-ups: Regular health check-ups can help identify and address any underlying health issues that may affect sexual health.

11. Avoid Performance Pressure: Putting too much pressure on sexual performance can lead to anxiety and performance-related issues. Focus on intimacy and emotional connection with your partner.

12. Seek Professional Help: If you experience persistent sexual health concerns, consult a healthcare provider or a specialist in men's sexual health.

6.2 Common Sexual Health Issues

Men may encounter various sexual health issues throughout their lives. It's essential to be aware of these concerns and seek appropriate support when needed. Here are some common sexual health issues men may face:

1. Erectile Dysfunction (ED): ED is the inability to achieve or maintain an erection sufficient for sexual intercourse. It can be caused by physical factors (e.g., diabetes, cardiovascular disease) or psychological factors (e.g., stress, anxiety).

2. Premature Ejaculation (PE): PE is when a man ejaculates before or shortly after penetration, often causing distress or

dissatisfaction for both partners.

3. Low Libido (Low Sex Drive): Low libido refers to a decreased interest in sexual activity. It can be influenced by hormonal imbalances, medications, stress, or relationship issues.

4. Performance Anxiety: Performance anxiety is the fear of not being able to perform sexually, leading to anxiety and potential difficulties in achieving or maintaining an erection.

5. Peyronie's Disease: Peyronie's disease involves the development of fibrous scar tissue inside the penis, leading to curvature or pain during erections.

6. Testosterone Deficiency: Low testosterone levels can affect sexual desire and function. It may lead to symptoms like fatigue, decreased muscle mass, and mood changes.

7. Sexually Transmitted Infections (STIs): Unprotected sexual activity can lead to the transmission of STIs, such as chlamydia, gonorrhea, herpes, and human papillomavirus (HPV).

8. Prostate Health Issues: Prostate conditions like benign prostatic hyperplasia (BPH) and prostate cancer can impact urinary and sexual function.

9. Delayed Ejaculation: Delayed ejaculation refers to difficulty or delay in reaching orgasm or

ejaculation during sexual
activity.

10. Infertility: Male infertility can
be caused by various factors,
including low sperm count,
poor sperm motility, or
blockages in the reproductive
system.

If you experience any sexual health
issues that persist or cause distress,
don't hesitate to seek professional
help. Qualified healthcare providers
can provide appropriate assessments,
diagnoses, and treatments to address
sexual health concerns effectively.

CHAPTER 7

Building Healthy Habits

Building healthy habits is essential for maintaining overall health and well-being. Consistency and sustainability are key to making positive lifestyle changes. Here are some tips for creating a sustainable exercise routine and forming healthy eating habits:

7.1 Creating a Sustainable Exercise Routine

1. Start Slow and Gradual: If you're new to exercise or

getting back into it after a break, start with low-impact activities and gradually increase the intensity and duration. This approach reduces the risk of injury and burnout.

2. Choose Activities You Enjoy: Find physical activities that you genuinely enjoy. Whether it's dancing, hiking, swimming, cycling, or playing a sport, doing something you love makes it more likely that you'll stick with it.

3. Set Realistic Goals: Set achievable and realistic fitness goals. Focus on small milestones and celebrate your progress along the way.

4. Schedule Regular Workouts: Plan your exercise sessions and

incorporate them into your daily or weekly routine. Consistency is key to building a sustainable habit.

5. Mix It Up: Avoid doing the same workout every day. Variety not only keeps things interesting but also challenges different muscle groups and prevents plateaus.

6. Listen to Your Body: Pay attention to how your body feels during and after exercise. Rest when needed and modify your routine to suit your fitness level.

7. Incorporate Strength Training: Include strength training exercises in your routine to build muscle, improve bone density, and boost metabolism.

8. Seek Support and Accountability: Exercise with a friend, join a fitness class, or hire a personal trainer to stay motivated and accountable.

9. Embrace Active Living: Look for opportunities to be active throughout your day. Take the stairs, walk or bike instead of driving short distances, and incorporate physical activity into your leisure time.

10. Focus on Long-Term Health: Remember that fitness is a journey, not a destination. Aim to improve your overall health and well-being, rather than solely focusing on appearance or short-term goals.

7.2 Forming Healthy Eating Habits

1. Eat Balanced Meals: Aim to include a variety of nutrients in your meals, such as fruits, vegetables, whole grains, lean proteins, and healthy fats.

2. Portion Control: Pay attention to portion sizes to avoid overeating. Listen to your body's hunger and fullness cues.

3. Eat Mindfully: Avoid distractions while eating, and savor each bite. Mindful eating can help you become more aware of your food choices and prevent overeating.

4. Plan Your Meals: Plan your meals ahead of time to make

healthier choices and avoid impulsive, less nutritious options.

5. Hydrate: Drink plenty of water throughout the day. Sometimes, feelings of hunger are actually signs of thirst.

6. Limit Processed Foods: Minimize your intake of processed foods, which are often high in added sugars, unhealthy fats, and sodium.

7. Cook at Home: Cooking your meals at home gives you more control over ingredients and helps you make healthier choices.

8. Practice Moderation: Allow yourself occasional treats and indulgences without guilt.

Balance is key to forming sustainable eating habits.

9. Be Mindful of Emotional Eating: Identify triggers for emotional eating and find alternative ways to cope with emotions, such as exercise, journaling, or talking to a friend.

10. Seek Professional Guidance: If you have specific dietary needs or health concerns, consult a registered dietitian or healthcare provider for personalized nutrition advice.

Building healthy habits takes time and patience, so be kind to yourself throughout the process. Focus on progress, not perfection, and remember that small, consistent changes can lead to significant improvements in your overall health and well-being.

7.3 Incorporating Stress-Relief Techniques into Daily Life

Incorporating stress-relief techniques into daily life is crucial for promoting overall well-being and managing the challenges of modern living. Chronic stress can have negative effects on both physical and mental health, but practicing regular stress-relief techniques can help reduce its impact. Here are some effective stress-relief techniques that can be easily incorporated into your daily routine:

1. Mindfulness Meditation: Practice mindfulness meditation to focus on the

present moment without judgment. Spend a few minutes each day sitting quietly and observing your thoughts and sensations without getting carried away by them.

2. Deep Breathing Exercises: Engage in deep breathing exercises to activate the body's relaxation response. Take slow, deep breaths, hold for a few seconds, and then exhale slowly. This simple technique can be done anytime, anywhere.

3. Physical Activity: Regular exercise is a natural stress reliever. Engage in activities you enjoy, such as walking, jogging, yoga, or dancing, to release tension and boost mood-enhancing endorphins.

4. Time in Nature: Spend time outdoors in nature, whether it's a short walk in the park, gardening, or simply sitting under a tree. Nature has a calming effect on the mind and can help reduce stress.

5. Creative Outlets: Engage in creative activities like drawing, painting, writing, or crafting. Creative expression can be a cathartic and relaxing way to relieve stress.

6. Social Connections: Maintain and nurture your social connections. Spending time with friends and loved ones can provide emotional support and reduce feelings of stress and isolation.

7. Laughter Therapy: Laughing can be a powerful stress buster. Watch a funny movie, read a humorous book, or spend time with people who make you laugh.

8. Limit Screen Time: Take breaks from screens, including smartphones, computers, and TVs. Constant exposure to screens can contribute to stress and anxiety.

9. Mindful Eating: Practice mindful eating by savoring each bite and being fully present during meals. Avoid distractions and listen to your body's hunger and fullness cues.

10. Gratitude Practice: Cultivate gratitude by reflecting on the

positive aspects of your life.
Keep a gratitude journal and
write down things you are
thankful for each day.

11. Progressive Muscle Relaxation:
Practice progressive muscle
relaxation to release tension
from different muscle groups in
your body. Tense and then
relax each muscle group to
promote relaxation.

12. Establish Boundaries: Learn to
say no to additional
commitments when you feel
overwhelmed. Setting healthy
boundaries protects your time
and energy.

Remember that not every technique
works for everyone, so experiment
with different stress-relief techniques
to find what suits you best. Integrating

these practices into your daily life can help you better manage stress, promote relaxation, and enhance your overall well-being. It's essential to prioritize self-care and make time for stress relief, as this investment in yourself will contribute to a healthier and happier life.

CHAPTER 8

Weight Management

Weight management is essential for maintaining overall health and well-being. Understanding body mass index (BMI), adopting healthy approaches to weight loss or gain, and balancing caloric intake and expenditure are crucial aspects of effective weight management.

8.1 Understanding Body Mass Index (BMI)

Body Mass Index (BMI) is a measure used to assess whether a person's weight is within a healthy range based on their height. It is calculated by dividing an individual's weight in kilograms by the square of their height in meters (BMI = weight in kg / height in m²). BMI provides a general indication of whether a person is underweight, normal weight, overweight, or obese. Here are the BMI classifications:

- Underweight: BMI less than 18.5

- Normal Weight: BMI 18.5 to 24.9

- Overweight: BMI 25 to 29.9

- Obese: BMI 30 or higher

While BMI is a useful screening tool, it does not directly measure body fat or consider individual variations in body composition, such as muscle mass. Therefore, it is essential to interpret BMI results in combination with other factors, such as waist circumference and overall health.

8.2 Healthy Approaches to Weight Loss or Gain

Weight loss or gain should be approached in a healthy and sustainable manner. Extreme dieting or crash diets are not recommended, as they can be harmful to overall health and lead to temporary results. Instead, consider the following healthy approaches:

For Weight Loss:

- Set Realistic Goals: Aim for a gradual weight loss of 0.5 to 1 kg (1 to 2 pounds) per week to ensure it is sustainable.

- **Balanced Diet:** Focus on a balanced diet that includes a variety of nutrient-dense foods, such as fruits, vegetables, whole grains, lean proteins, and healthy fats.

- **Portion Control:** Pay attention to portion sizes to avoid overeating.

- **Regular Exercise:** Incorporate regular physical activity into your routine to burn calories and improve overall health.

- **Stay Hydrated:** Drink plenty of water throughout the day to support weight loss efforts.

- **Mindful Eating:** Eat mindfully and pay attention to hunger and fullness cues.

For Weight Gain:

- Healthy Calories: Choose nutrient-rich foods that provide additional calories and nutrition, such as nuts, seeds, avocados, and healthy oils.

- Strength Training: Engage in resistance training to build muscle mass and support healthy weight gain.

- Balanced Diet: Ensure your diet includes a balance of macronutrients (carbohydrates, proteins, and fats) and micronutrients (vitamins and minerals).

- Regular Meals and Snacks: Avoid skipping meals and aim to have regular, balanced meals and snacks throughout the day.

8.3 Balancing Caloric Intake and Expenditure

Balancing caloric intake and expenditure is crucial for weight management. To maintain weight, calories consumed should be equal to calories expended. To lose weight, create a calorie deficit by consuming fewer calories than you burn. To gain weight, create a calorie surplus by consuming more calories than you burn. Here are some tips to achieve balance:

- Track Caloric Intake: Keep a food journal or use a calorie tracking app to monitor your daily caloric intake.

- Estimate Caloric Expenditure: Use tools or calculators to estimate your daily caloric expenditure based on factors

like age, gender, weight, and
activity level.

- Portion Control: Be mindful of portion sizes and avoid overeating.

- Stay Active: Engage in regular physical activity to burn calories and support weight management goals.

Individual needs and circumstances vary, so it's essential to consult with a healthcare provider or a registered dietitian for personalized advice and guidance on weight management. A healthy approach to weight management focuses on overall well-being and is sustainable in the long term.

CHAPTER 9

Maintaining Motivation and Overcoming Challenges

9.1 Staying Consistent with Your Health Goals

Staying consistent with your health goals is key to achieving long-term success. Here are some strategies to help you stay motivated and committed to your goals:

1. Set Realistic Goals: Set achievable and specific goals that align with your abilities and lifestyle. Break larger goals

into smaller, manageable steps to track your progress.

2. Find Intrinsic Motivation: Identify your personal reasons for pursuing your health goals. Connect with the intrinsic benefits, such as improved energy, mood, and overall well-being.

3. Create a Routine: Establish a daily or weekly routine that includes healthy habits, exercise, and self-care activities. Consistency breeds success.

4. Track Your Progress: Keep a journal or use apps to track your progress. Celebrate small victories and use setbacks as learning opportunities.

5. Reward Yourself: Celebrate
    your achievements with non-
    food rewards, such as treating
    yourself to a spa day or buying
    something you've wanted for a
    while.

6. Surround Yourself with
    Positivity: Surround yourself
    with supportive and
    encouraging people who share
    similar health goals. Their
    positive influence can keep you
    motivated.

7. Visualize Success: Visualize
    yourself achieving your health
    goals and the positive impact it
    will have on your life.
    Visualization can reinforce
    your commitment.

8. Be Flexible: Understand that
    life can be unpredictable. If you

miss a workout or make an unhealthy choice, don't dwell on it. Get back on track and focus on the next opportunity to make healthier choices.

9.2 Dealing with Plateaus and Setbacks

Plateaus and setbacks are normal in any journey towards better health. Here's how to handle them:

1. Stay Patient: Plateaus are a natural part of progress. Be patient and continue to put in effort; results will come.

2. Reevaluate Your Approach: Assess your current strategies and consider making adjustments. It may be time to

change up your workout routine
or reassess your nutrition plan.

3. Set New Challenges: Push
   yourself to try new exercises or
   set new fitness targets.
   Introducing variety can reignite
   your motivation.

4. Seek Support: Share your
   struggles with supportive
   friends, family, or online
   communities. Often, others
   have experienced similar
   challenges and can offer advice
   and encouragement.

5. Embrace Setbacks as Learning
   Opportunities: Understand that
   setbacks happen to everyone.
   Use them as opportunities to
   learn and grow from the
   experience.

6. Focus on Non-Scale Victories:
    Look beyond the scale and
    focus on other positive
    changes, such as increased
    energy, improved sleep, or
    enhanced mood.

9.3 Finding Support and Accountability

Having support and accountability
can significantly impact your
motivation and success. Here's how to
find it:

1. Enlist a Workout Buddy:
    Partner with a friend or family
    member who shares your health
    goals. Exercising together can
    make workouts more enjoyable
    and create a sense of
    accountability.

2. Join Fitness Classes or Groups: Participate in group fitness classes or activities. The camaraderie and encouragement from fellow participants can be motivating.

3. Hire a Personal Trainer or Coach: A qualified professional can provide personalized guidance, create a tailored workout plan, and keep you accountable.

4. Use Online Resources: Join online forums, fitness apps, or social media groups dedicated to health and fitness. You can connect with like-minded individuals and find support virtually.

5. Seek Professional Guidance: Consult with a healthcare

provider, registered dietitian, or mental health professional if you need personalized support or face specific challenges.

CHAPTER 10

Aging Gracefully

10.1 Health Considerations as You Age

As we age, certain health considerations become more important. Here are some key areas to focus on:

1. Regular Health Check-ups: Schedule regular check-ups with healthcare providers to monitor your overall health, manage chronic conditions, and address any age-related concerns.

2. Maintain a Healthy Diet:
    Emphasize nutrient-dense foods
    and stay hydrated. Adequate
    calcium and vitamin D intake is
    essential for bone health.

3. Physical Activity: Stay active
    with regular exercise to
    maintain strength, flexibility,
    and balance. Activities like
    walking, swimming, and yoga
    are beneficial.

4. Cognitive Health: Engage in
    mentally stimulating activities
    to support brain health, such as
    puzzles, reading, or learning
    new skills.

5. Preventive Health Measures:
    Stay up-to-date on
    vaccinations, cancer screenings,
    and other preventive measures

to catch potential health issues
early.

10.2 Promoting Longevity and Quality of Life

Promote longevity and enhance your quality of life with the following practices:

1. Manage Stress: Practice stress-reduction techniques like meditation, mindfulness, or relaxation exercises to improve overall well-being.

2. Social Connections: Maintain social interactions and strong relationships with friends, family, and community to combat feelings of isolation.

3. Maintain Mental Health: Address mental health concerns promptly, seeking support from mental health professionals when needed.

4. Avoid Harmful Habits: Limit alcohol consumption, avoid smoking or substance abuse, and practice safe behaviors to protect your health.

5. Stay Curious and Engaged: Keep learning, pursue hobbies, and engage in activities that bring joy and fulfillment.

10.3 Embracing Lifestyle Adjustments

As you age, lifestyle adjustments may be necessary. Embrace these changes with a positive outlook:

1. Adapt Exercise Routines:
   Modify exercise routines to suit
   your changing abilities and
   preferences. Focus on low-
   impact activities that support
   joint health.

2. Balanced Nutrition: Adjust
   your diet to meet changing
   nutrient needs, considering
   factors like metabolism,
   digestion, and dental health.

3. Sleep Quality: Prioritize
   sufficient and restful sleep to
   support overall health and
   energy levels.

4. Safety Measures: Take
   precautions to prevent falls and
   injuries, such as using handrails
   and maintaining a clutter-free
   living space.

5. Seek Support: Don't hesitate to seek support from family, friends, or professionals as you navigate the aging process.

Aging gracefully is about maintaining your health, independence, and vitality as you grow older. Embrace the journey, celebrate each stage of life, and make choices that prioritize your well-being and happiness.